P9-DFX-456

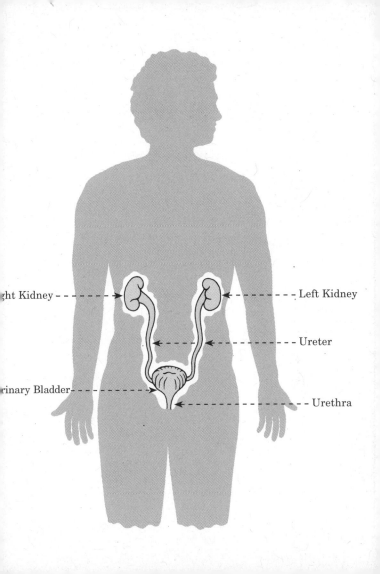

ght Kidney - - - - - - - → ← - - - - - - Left Kidney

← - - - - - - - - Ureter

rinary Bladder - - - - - - → ← - - - - - - - - Urethra

What's My Pee

Authors of the #2 best-seller
What's Your Poo Telling You?

**By Josh Richman and
Anish Sheth, M.D.**

Illustrations by Matt Johnstone

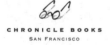

CHRONICLE BOOKS
SAN FRANCISCO

Telling Me?

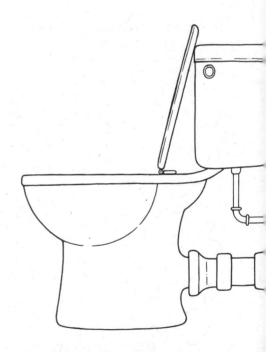

Library of Congress Cataloging-in-Publication Data:

Richman, Josh.
    "What's my pee telling me?" / Josh Richman and Anish Sheth.
      p. cm.
    ISBN 978-0-8118-6877-8
    1. Urine—Popular works. 2. Feces—Popular works. 3. Flatulence—Popular works. 4. Bezoars—Popular works. 5. Medicine—Miscellanea. I. Sheth, Anish. II. Title.

QP211.R53 2009
612.4'61—dc22

                                        2009010936

Manufactured in Canada

Designed by Jacob T. Gardner
Typeset in New Century Schoolbook and Cooper Black

Bubblicious is a registered trademark of Cadbury Adams USA LLC.
Coca-Cola is a registered trademark of The Coca-Cola Company.
Dubble Bubble is a registered trademark of Concord Brands.
Pepto-Bismol is a registered trademark of The Procter & Gamble Company.
Pyridium is a registered trademark of Warner Chilcott Company, Inc.
Stickum is a trademark of Mueller Sports Medicine.

10 9 8 7 6 5 4 3

Chronicle Books LLC
680 Second Street
San Francisco, CA 94107
www.chroniclebooks.com

Acknowledgments

To our families and friends for their continued support of our quest for poo-phoria.

To Samantha, Rohan, and Ria for continuing to provide inspiration that goes well beyond daily diaper changes.

CONTENTS

Chapter Four: Bodily Myths Exploded

Myth or Truth?

Introduction

We couldn't hold it in any longer. This is one sequel that just had to be written. Yes, here it is, book number two featuring good ol' number one, plus loads more. Our initial foray into the world of dookie, *What's Your Poo Telling You?*, broke the seal of secrecy on this most fascinating of subjects. Now it is time for the movement to continue.

What's My Pee Telling Me? continues our quest to demystify the inner workings of the human body through discussion of what comes out of it. Besides poo and its closely related byproduct, flatulence, this digest ventures into unchartered waters, plunging wholeheartedly into urine, the oft-forgotten member of the excreta empire. *What's My Pee Telling Me?* furthers the belief that each bodily emission—solid, liquid, or gaseous—can offer valuable information about our health.

The time has come once again to embrace what escapes us unnoticed and to explode some myths about bodily functions. So grab your book, sit down on the best seat in the house, and enjoy!

Chapter One:

What's My Pee Telling Me?

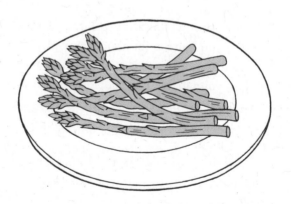

While it's rare to hear someone announce that they need to poo or fart, it's quite common to hear a friend exclaim, "I'm going to go take a leak," or "I need to pee before we leave." Unfortunately, this openness has not translated into a greater understanding of what pee can tell us about our health.

Although we call it number one, pee has long been number two, unfairly in line behind poo when it comes to discussion of our bodily waste. Urine is too often regarded as uninteresting, lacking the cachet of poo, too often dismissed as nothing more than yellow-tinged liquid. However, not only can you learn a lot about your physical well-being through awareness of the look, feel, and smell of your urine, but pee, more so than poo, lends itself to easy examination. Pee can even be seen as it emerges from the body, though this is easier for men.

Through discussion of urine's impressive array of colors, quantities, and smells (aah, asparagus), we shed light on pee's ability to teach us about our health. Whether you're sitting or standing, the time has come for pee to make a splash.

Pungent Pee

Synonyms: *Smelly Stream, Asparagus Aftershock, Scrambled Eggs*

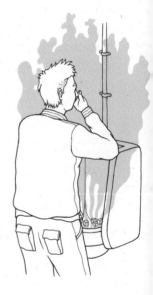

In most instances, freshly produced pee is remarkably odorless. (A pee puddle that has been sitting around for a few hours is a different story altogether.) In the rare case where fresh urine has a detectable aroma, it usually takes one of two forms: fruity or eggy. The latter stench most notoriously occurs after eating asparagus and can take pee-ers (and those in the immediate vicinity) by surprise. Pungent Pee has been invoked by some as the sole reason to employ a courtesy flush while going number one.

Dr. Stool says: By far the most famous of pee fragrances is asparagus aroma. This foul, eggy odor results from the release of sulfur-containing compounds during asparagus digestion. These compounds are absorbed from the digestive tract into the bloodstream and then filtered into urine by the kidneys. Amazingly, asparagus aroma can be detected in urine within fifteen minutes of consuming asparagus! However, it turns out that only 50 percent of the world's population has ever experienced the aroma of asparagus pee. Initially, this was thought to be due to differences in the way some of us digested asparagus, but now it is believed that while all of us excrete these sulfur-containing compounds in our urine, only 50 percent of us have the genes needed to detect their smell. A tip: If you cut off asparagus tips prior to consumption, you won't get Pungent Pee.

Driblets

If you're a frequent flusher with fruity-smelling urine, you may want to get tested for diabetes. High blood sugar causes changes in the way the body generates energy. One of the by-products is a class of molecules called ketones, which spill into the urine and give it a fresh berry-type aroma. You may also find yourself going more often, as the body tries to expel excess glucose through urination.

Mellow Yellow

Synonyms: *Gold Rush, Sunny P*

No color may have more positive associations than yellow. Yellow sunflowers are widely considered to be some of the most cheerful flowers on earth. The yellow jersey represents victory in the Tour de France. Yellow smiley faces are the symbol of happiness. And, yes, urine, too, has always been associated with the color yellow. Urinophiles love to wax poetic about pee's sparkling, golden appearance—seventeenth-century alchemists were convinced that the yellow color was due to the presence of gold in urine. While a yellow-tinged hue to urine is normal, darker, richer yellows are less desirable. In the world of pee, bolder is *not* better: mellow yellow is the way to go.

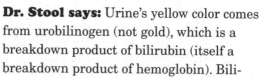 **Dr. Stool says:** Urine's yellow color comes from urobilinogen (not gold), which is a breakdown product of bilirubin (itself a breakdown product of hemoglobin). Bilirubin enters the kidneys where it is converted to yellow-hued urobilins and excreted in the urine.

Assuming normal levels of urobilins, the color intensity of urine is determined simply by the amount of water passing through the kidneys.

Dehydration causes the kidneys to retain water for the body's use, so less water ends up being excreted into the urinary stream, thereby concentrating urobilins and rendering urine a darker color. Simple tests can measure the concentration of urine by assessing something called the specific gravity. In general, the higher the specific gravity, the darker the urine will appear. In fact, urine color can be used as a rough gauge of the body's hydration status during episodes of food poisoning or after a long-distance run. Dark yellow urine indicates concentrated urine, signaling the need to consume more water.

Driblets

The ideal urine color has been likened to a pale lemonade.

CRYSTAL CLEAR

Sometimes after a tinkle, you may glance into the toilet only to see a bowl of crystal clear water, leaving you to wonder, "Where did my yellow go?" Clear pee reflects an excess of water in the urine. This dilutes the concentration of urobilinogen and makes urine seem like nothing more than lukewarm H_2O. The most likely explanation for clear urine is the consumption of large amounts of water. Our urine tends to be darkest when we wake up (our kidneys retain water to keep our bodies hydrated at night) and progressively lightens as we replenish our water stores. In general, clear urine is a positive sign telling you that you are well hydrated.

Clear urine can also be one of the first signs that you are well on the path toward inebriation. Within twenty minutes of your first alcoholic beverage, the body's level of anti-diuretic hormone (ADH) decreases. This hormone normally functions to *prevent* urination and allows the body to conserve water. As you continue to toss back drink after drink, levels of ADH in the body plummet, effectively making the kidneys nothing more than conduits for the massive amounts of liquid you are ingesting. The end result is large amounts of dilute urine, which leads to dehydration, hangovers, and the well-known admonition against "breaking the seal."

Red Rum

Synonyms: *Uh Oh Go, Red Rain, Bloody Mary*

Peeing red can turn your toilet into an unwelcome bowl of fruit punch. As urination progresses, the toilet water begins to turn from a mildly worrisome shade of pink into an ominous crimson. Often the appearance of red toilet water can be a source of confusion. Females often wonder whether their menstrual cycle has come early. Men and women alike have difficulty determining the origin of bleeding in instances when pee and poo are deposited simultaneously.

 Dr. Stool says: Red urine is almost always a sign of bleeding in the urinary tract. Hematuria, as it is called, is most commonly seen in urinary tract infections affecting the bladder and kidneys. This bleeding is mild and can be associated with burning (see "The Flame Thrower," page 23). Bleeding can also be seen in the presence of kidney stones (excruciating belly pain is usually the most prominent symptom), kidney inflammation, bruised kidneys from being punched or tackled, and cancers of the urinary tract (prostate, bladder, etc.).

Occasionally, red urine can be seen after strenuous activity such as running a marathon. In this case, repeated trauma to the soles of the feet is thought to cause damage to red blood cells which travel through small, fragile capillaries, thereby releasing hemoglobin into the bloodstream. When large amounts of hemoglobin are released, some of it is filtered in the kidneys and makes its way into the urine. This phenomenon was first noticed in army recruits after long marches and has come to be known as "march hemoglobinuria."

Thankfully, bleeding is not the only cause of red urine. Consuming large amounts of beets and rhubarb can also turn the urine red. If this is the cause, the urine should quickly return to a normal color (assuming you have stopped eating the offending food).

Final word: While you should contact your doctor at the first sign of red urine, it is important not to overreact. Keep in mind the principle of food coloring—just a few drops will dramatically alter the color of even a large bucket of water.

Porphyria, believed by some to explain the erratic behavior of King George III, is caused by defective enzymes involved in making heme (a component of hemoglobin). Diagnosis of this rare disease can be made by observing a fresh urine specimen turn from yellow to red when exposed to sunlight.

PISS LIKE A RACE HORSE

The saying "I have to piss like a racehorse" has made its way into modern vernacular without many understanding its origin. Horses produce 1.5 to 2 gallons of urine daily (by comparison, an adult human male makes 1 to 2 quarts per day). But race horses don't pee any more than other horses. There appear to be two common explanations for this phrase's derivation:

(1) The observation that racehorses pee exorbitant amounts at a time may be due to the fact that they dislike peeing outside of their stables. A racehorse will hold its urine and stifle the extreme urge to pee until they are back in the safe confines of their pens.

(2) Some say this phrase originated with the practice of giving diuretics to racehorses before a race (Performance-Enhancing Pee!)

Vitamin Water

Synonyms: *B Pee, Vitamin P, Liquid Highlighter*

While the normal palette of pee can range from completely clear to bright yellow, there are times when pee comes out a fluorescent yellow, or even a bright orange. The seemingly unnatural vibrancy makes this the most dramatic of pee's color variations—its brightness can leave you searching for the nearest pair of sunglasses. Some people are tempted to turn off the lights and see whether the toilet water glows in the dark. When you experience Vitamin Water pee, you may start to wonder if your diet has included antifreeze or highlighter ink.

 Dr. Stool says: Bright yellow or orange urine is virtually always caused by the ingestion of vitamins and medications. Somehow, it just makes sense that fluorescent urine wouldn't occur as a result of any naturally occurring bodily process. Vitamin B supplementation has become popular due to its potential to boost the immune system and to promote healthier skin. When taken in large doses, the body

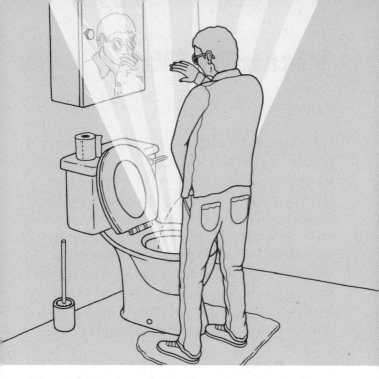

disposes of the excess vitamins in the urine, lending it a bright yellow/orange color. Other medications including Senna (used to treat constipation) and Pyridium (interestingly, used in treatment of urinary tract infections) are well-known culprits of orange-hued urine. The change in urine color is not harmful in any way, but may be a sign that you are taking more vitamins than your body needs.

WATER REQUIREMENTS

The answer to how much water we need to drink per day comes from first determining how much water we have lost. If we assume a normal day's activity (i.e., no marathon), it turns out the numbers are pretty constant.

Our water losses:

Urine	1.5 liters
Breathing/Poo/Sweat	1.0 liter
Total	2.5 liters/day

Assuming we take in half a liter of water per day just by eating a normal diet, the average person needs two liters of water per day—about eight glasses.

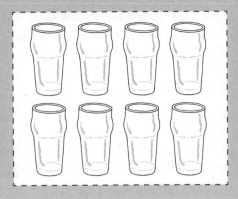

The Flame Thrower

Synonyms: *Fire Water; Painful Pee; Tamale Tinkle; Yes, Yes, No!*

Burn, baby, burn. There may be variations in this pee's color and frequency, but its most distinguishing feature is the excruciating, spine-chilling burn felt during its expulsion. The Flame Thrower will leave you gripping the handicapped rail, as every drop of urine released is matched by an almost equal amount of perspiration flowing down your forehead. This sensation of peeing out grains of sand or cayenne pepper can drive someone to stop drinking fluids altogether to avoid the agony of further trips to the bathroom.

 Dr. Stool says: Few men have ever experienced the Flame Thrower, while virtually all women have (some on multiple occasions). Owing to their shorter urethra, women are more likely to develop urinary tract infections, most commonly involving the bladder.

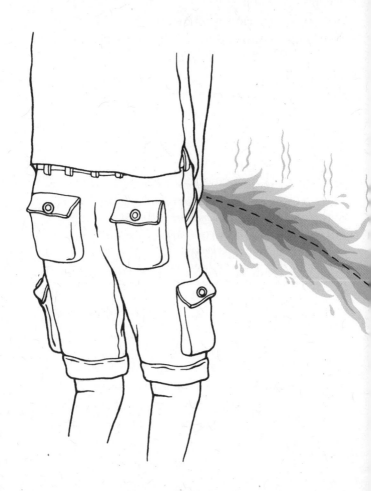

The presence of bacteria in the normally sterile urinary system causes inflammation and leads to a burning sensation during voiding. Urine can also turn bloody and come at more frequent intervals (inflammation causes irritation of the bladder and the urge to go more often). Thankfully, treatment with antibiotics is curative.

Driblets

Women plagued by recurrent urinary infections may want to consider downing a glass of cranberry juice every now and then. Several studies have shown that a specific compound, proanthocyanidin, found in cranberry juice, prevents bacteria like E. coli from attaching to the urinary tract and causing infections. Not a fan of cranberry juice? Turns out blueberry juice may work just as well, if you can find it.

Bubble Bath

Synonyms: *Foamy Flow; Jet Stream; Peecuzzi*

Okay, so what guy hasn't played that game where you try to cover the entire surface of the toilet bowl with air bubbles while you pee? Bubbles are created by the turbulence resulting from urine hitting the water. In general, the faster the urinary stream, the more bubbles it creates. But in some cases, pee takes on a foamy appearance all on its own, turning your toilet into an unexpected bubble bath, and causing you, for a split second, to consider grabbing your rubber ducky and a loofah.

 Dr. Stool says: Foamy urine can be caused by turbulent urination or can be a sign of proteins in the urine (proteinuria). Proteins are useful building blocks for our cells and thus are kept in the body by the kidneys' filtration system. When this filtration system becomes damaged (most commonly by diabetes or hypertension), protein molecules normally kept out of the urinary stream are allowed to enter. A simple test performed on a urine specimen is a quick way to check for excessive protein.

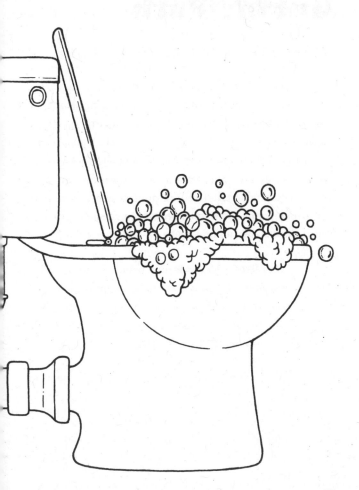

Gravy Train

Synonyms: *Brown Bonanza, Chocolate Drizzle, The Coca-Cola*

When seeing brown urine for the first time, you may attribute the toilet water discoloration to an ineffective flush following a bowel movement. As you begin to curse your roommate for not monitoring the toilet bowl for poo remnants, you glance down and notice a distinct cola-like quality to the urinary stream as it emerges from your body. The Gravy Train makes one wonder whether it's possible to pee out poop.

Dr. Stool says: Occasionally, it may seem as if the body has its signals crossed, turning urine brown and stool white. Brown pee is caused by liver dysfunction or a blockage in the bile ducts that causes spilling of bile into the bloodstream and then into the urine. Bile lends urine a dark greenish-brown color, classically described as being "Coca-Cola-colored" or "tea-colored" in appearance. Blockage of the bile duct caused by a gallstone also prevents bile from entering the intestinal tract, thereby depriving stool of its usual chocolate color. Because bile duct blockage can also result from pancreatic tumors, the combination of dark urine and pale-colored stools should always prompt a visit to the doctor.

Driblets

The Koryak people of Siberia drink urine in conjunction with their ceremonial use of psychedelic mushrooms. The active alkaloids of the mushrooms remain unchanged as they pass through the human body a second time, allowing the urine to retain the intoxicating effects of the mushroom.

Pee-phoria

Synonyms: *Pleasure Pee, Piss Bliss, Ecstasy Pee*

Sometimes we are forced to hold in pee, typically on a long car ride or in an important meeting. What begins as a small urge rapidly becomes an unbearable discomfort, with each bump in the road serving as a reminder of your overloaded bladder. When finally able to stand and head for the toilet, some will engage in what is commonly referred to as the "Pee Pee Dance" or "Tee Tee Tango," a series of random body gyrations that may include swaying back and forth, bending over and standing up, even hopping up and down (although this seems counter-productive) before the eventual release of pee. As urine begins to flow, this agony gives way to utter elation. Some have described a cool, tingling sensation that radiates throughout the body as the urine is discharged.

 Dr. Stool says: Pee-phoria results from stimulation of nerve endings in the urinary system that lend a sense of sublime relaxation. Furthermore, there is a sense of relief as bladder pressure diminishes, leaving you feeling light on your feet. In most cases, there is no danger in holding in urine for a short while. Pee-phoria's intensity is directly proportional to the degree of agony experienced while holding it in.

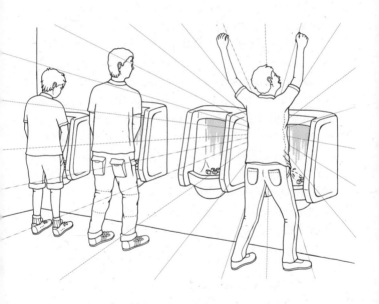

PERFORMANCE-ENHANCING PEE

While some baseball players fear the discussion of pee, thinking that a drug test is soon to follow, there are some who harness the power of pee to boost on-field performance. Several major leaguers, including Moises Alou and Jorge Posada, forego batting gloves and pee on their hands to prevent and relieve calluses. Similarly, heavyweight boxing champ Vitali Klitschko uses an old Ukranian secret passed down to him by his grandmother to keep his hands from swelling up like other boxers' hands. Yes, he wraps his hands in his infant's diapers before a match.

These athletes have figured out what urine therapy believers have been saying for centuries—massaging your skin with urine can keep it healthy and soft. The dermatologic benefits of urine are largely due to urea, a substance that can be also be found in many commercially available lotions. Although urine is sterile, Dr. Stool feels obligated to recommend that batboys wear gloves at all times and that you avoid shaking hands with Klitschko.

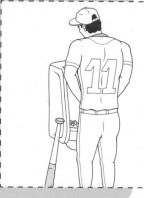

The Drip

Synonyms: *Prostate Pee, Faulty Fountain, Sputtering Hose*

Men: To the list of things that slow down as you age, add the speed of your urine stream. As young boys, we engaged in distance-peeing contests, shamelessly flaunting our ability to forcefully propel our urine long distances. Almost universally, this once-robust jet stream will eventually give way to frustrating drips and drabs more akin to a leaky faucet than a fire hose. Despite forceful straining and the occasional milking maneuver, urinary flow can deteriorate to the point of complete obstruction. The inability to satisfactorily empty the bladder leads to frequent, frustrating trips to the bathroom and multiple nighttime awakenings to visit the loo.

 Dr. Stool says: Normal urinary flow is a function of the strength of bladder contraction versus the degree of flow resistance in the urethra. Normal urinary flow rate is dependent on age and gender but typically ranges from ten to twenty milliliters per second. Enlargement of the prostate gland, a normally walnut-sized structure which encircles the urethra, is a nearly universal occurrence as men age. The enlarged gland can compress the urethra and cause an increased resistance to urinary flow, thereby decreasing urinary stream velocity. Mild cases of prostatic hypertrophy can be treated with medicines that shrink the gland. More severe cases can cause complete obstruction to urinary flow, necessitating the surgical placement of a urinary catheter.

Doo You Know
Men pee faster than women up until the age of fifty or so, when women take the lead.

STAGE FRIGHT

Stage fright has plagued mankind since we began peeing in the company of others. The typical stage fright scenario occurs at a ballpark or other places where herds of men pee in small confined spaces. Pee Anxiety, colloquially known as Tinkle Terror or Ballpark Bladder, and scientifically known as paruresis, or Shy Bladder Syndrome, is surprisingly common, with 7–10 percent of American men reporting difficulty urinating in close proximity to others. For a majority of paruresis suffers, the issue is psychological, a form of anxiety that typically begins in the teenage years and may stem from embarrassment at having the genital region exposed.

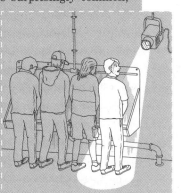

In older men, alcoholic beverages can cause an already enlarged prostate gland to swell, causing obstruction to urine flowing out of the bladder.

Pebble Pee

Synonyms: *Tortured Tinkle, Agony Pee*

Yes, ladies, the passage of pebble pee is as excruciatingly painful as childbirth—without an epidural. More often occurring in men, Pebble Pee often begins as just another trip to the bathroom. The onset of sharp groin pain (similar to labor pains) is the first sign that things are about to get interesting. What usually follows is a several-hour-long melee filled with writhing, perspiration, and profanity. Only with the passage of the offending kidney stone does the agony end. Unlike the joyous results of pregnancy labor, the only fruit of your agony is a two-millimeter pebble resting tauntingly in the toilet bowl.

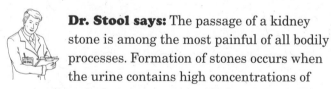 **Dr. Stool says:** The passage of a kidney stone is among the most painful of all bodily processes. Formation of stones occurs when the urine contains high concentrations of certain substances (most commonly calcium). These substances begin to precipitate and form crystals, which then coalesce to form stones. Stones can

become lodged anywhere along the urinary tract, causing excruciating pain as urine flow becomes blocked and muscles contract more forcibly in an attempt to overcome the obstruction. Depending on the site of obstruction, pain may be felt anywhere from the back to the groin to the urethra. Increasing urine flow by drinking large quantities of water and using pain medications are the usual treatments while awaiting spontaneous stone passage. In some cases, surgical intervention is needed to remove large stones too big to pass through the urethra.

WHY CAN'T MEN PEE STRAIGHT?

Since the invention of toilets, men have struggled to hit the mark. Men can shoot a basketball into a hoop from over twenty feet away and sink thirty-foot putts on the golf course, but give them a wide-open toilet bowl and a stream of urine and there is no telling where their liquid gold will end up. Things have been so bad for so long that women have given up on men's ability to control their pee, focusing their efforts instead on making sure men urinate with the toilet seat up, then insisting that they put the seat back down after they're finished.

The main difference between male and female urinary physics is that women need only pee in one direction (down) while men need to pee in both the horizontal and vertical directions. In order to cover the horizontal distance, urine must be expelled with enough force to make it to the toilet. Too little velocity and it ends up on the floor; too much and it could end up just about anywhere.

Most men have no trouble controlling their urine velocity in midstream, when velocity and trajectory are predictable and constant. The main problem occurs at the beginning and the end of urination, when their control over stream velocity is poor. Take the example of a garden hose: the first few spurts and last few spurts are unpredictable because the water molecules are moving turbulently and at different speeds. Once a smooth, laminar flow is achieved, the water molecules move in unison, and hence, more predictably.

So what is the solution? Short of sitting down (in essence, eliminating the need for urine to cover horizontal ground), one can try standing close to the toilet bowl and aiming downward much as possible. Not inclined to squat over the toilet? Just make sure to put the toilet seat up before you let loose.

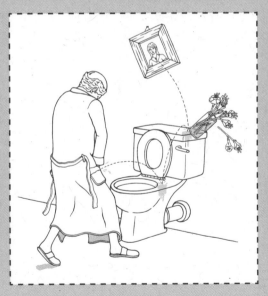

Chapter Two:

Poo Too!

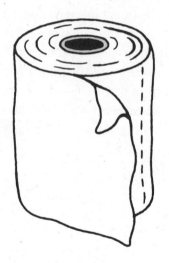

Regardless of the form, flow, or feeling generated by poo, a bowel movement is universally known as number two. It is only fitting, therefore, that the second chapter of our second book would revisit this topic—a double digest, if you will.

We wondered what more could be said about our beloved deuce. After extensive research, it turns out that *What's Your Poo Telling You?* only scratched the surface. Not unlike the proverbial iceberg, there is much more poo beneath the toilet waterline. In the following pages, you will not only find discussions of some rare poos, but a focus on how diet and the pressure to be thin affect the bottom line.

So sit back and relax. It is time for a second session of learning about what your poo is telling you!

Paradoxical Poo

Synonyms: *Crushing Combo, Excremental Dilemma*

When your constipation gets bad, you can go for days, maybe weeks, without much activity in the number two department. Finally, after much frustration, you may sense that you are on the precipice of a breakthrough and you enter the bathroom preparing to push out the responsible poo plug. However, instead of the free-flowing release of stool, you may be surprised when a spurt of brown liquid splatters mockingly into the toilet. Feeling that the lack of regular defecation has somehow affected your senses, you push again, which results in the expulsion of even more liquid stool. As the days go by, you find only temporary relief from the agony of the logjam through small bursts of unsatisfying, watery diarrhea. While you are glad to be free from total constipation, you are left unfulfilled, wondering when normal, solid stool will return. Is it possible to be constipated and have diarrhea at the same time?

Dr. Stool says: Seemingly flying in the face of poo logic, Paradoxical Poo is the experience of having constipation and diarrhea *at the same time*. Also called "overflow diarrhea," Paradoxical Poo occurs when watery stool leaks around an unyielding poo plug, a condition called fecal impaction. This ailment is characterized by the presence of a hard bolus of stool which literally plugs up the rectum and prevents passage of normal fecal material. While poo's egress from the body is impeded, liquid stool can seep around the edges and give the appearance of diarrhea, sometimes tricking physicians into prescribing medications that slow down the GI tract and worsen the underlying constipation. Once an accurate diagnosis is made, treatment is with laxatives and, if needed, manual extraction of the poo plug.

Nuggets

Volvulus, a cause of intestinal obstruction, can occur when the floppiest section of the colon, the sigmoid colon, twists upon itself and prevents passage of fecal material. The highest incidence of this is seen in India, Iran, Russia, and Brazil, countries which make up the so-called "volvulus belt."

Never-Ending Wipe Poo

Synonyms: *Stickum Stool, Double-Sided Deuce, Tar Turd, TP Thief*

While the delivery of this poo may go off without a hitch, the clean-up is another story. Eager to give your creation a quick glance, wipe, and be on with your day, this poo gets you hung up during the cleanup. The first signs of an impending problem appear during the first wipe when the toilet paper reveals a stickier–than–usual substance in a greater–than–expected quantity. The Never-Ending

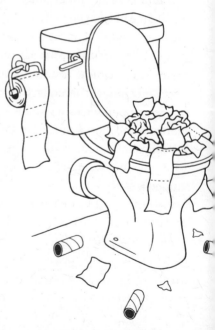

Wipe Poo (NEWP) has been likened to a dark maple syrup because of its typical dark color and viscous consistency. When repeated wipes continue to yield significant amounts of residual stool, you wonder if and when you will ever finish the cleanup. Frustrated, you may modify the wiping technique by increasing the force applied or by employing a bidirectional, back-and-forth maneuver. Alas, the problem may not be with the wiping technique or the quality of the toilet paper, but in the unique attributes of the poo.

 Dr. Stool says: The Never-Ending Wipe Poo can be caused by one of several factors. First, the stickier the poo, the more you will have to wipe. Usually by the time stool makes it to your rectum it is somewhat desiccated by the colon's avid absorption of water. However, if your stool passes quickly through the colon, there will be less time for absorption and your stool may have a more gel-like consistency.

High-viscosity stool can also occur when there is bleeding from stomach or small intestine. When blood mixes with stomach acid, it forms a black, tarry stool called melena. This mixture of blood and stool makes its way down the GI tract and produces a particularly sticky stool which resembles tar in color and consistency (its smell is also notably abhorrent). When a NEWP takes on this form, it could be a sign that blood loss is occurring from the stomach, most commonly due to a bleeding ulcer.

Another, thankfully more common, explanation for the NEWP is fecal contamination of large hemorrhoids. These engorged blood vessels may become soiled as stool passes through the anal canal and can be difficult to clean. This is especially true for large, prolapsing hemorrhoids which move in and out of the anal canal during a bowel movement.

A fourth cause of NEWP is the presence of a perianal fistula, an abnormal conduit between the inside of the intestines and the skin. This results in continuous passage of stool from the anal region, thereby mimicking the NEWP. This unfortunate condition is discussed under "Poobiquitous" (page 51).

The Life Raft

Synonyms: *The Safety Net, The Trifecta,*
The Poo Pillow

The mysterious practice of women traveling to
the bathroom in herds has resulted in one major
advance for mankind: the Life Raft. The Life Raft
arose, in large part, because of the need for women
to surreptitiously move their bowels in a public
bathroom. Traditional tactics to mask droppage

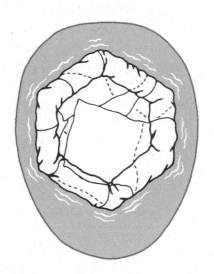

proved insufficient when in the proximity of five of your closest friends. Out of this necessity, the Life Raft was created—an ingenious innovation involving layering toilet paper in the toilet bowl *prior* to having a bowel movement in order to mask its sound. In fact, a properly executed Life Raft deployment results in "The Trifecta"—no noise, no splash, and no skidmark.

Dr. Stool says: The fear of backsplash has been around ever since people began dropping their deuces into a bowl of water. Small, dense particles of poo are at highest risk for causing a splash; this process is classically referred to as "buckshot." In reality, backsplash contamination, even from the grimiest of public toilets, is unlikely to cause serious health consequences. The Life Raft can help conceal poo's landing, but the only surefire way to prevent a splash of contaminated toilet water is to ensure the delivery of a single, lengthy bolus which effortlessly slides into place at the bottom of the toilet bowl. So to avoid embarrassing buckshot in front of your friends, eat lots of fiber and stay well hydrated!

GETTING THE JOB DONE

Work poo is a necessity for most. Unless you are unbelievably constipated or work three hours a day, you will probably be faced with the prospect of having to unload a work poo at one time or another. Some will attempt to avoid it at all costs while others will embrace it, even going as far as inserting a "bowel break" into their daily schedule. You should know, however, that there is a different set of rules when it comes to work poo. Failure to follow them is sure to result in a career-threatening walk of shame back to your desk.

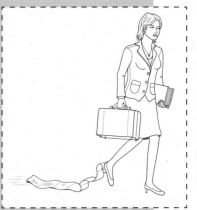

(1) Whenever possible, opt for a single-stall bathroom. A private bathroom in a different part of the office building is ideal. If you are fortunate enough to find a private bathroom, make sure there is absolutely no odor (or residual streak, for that matter) when you leave (there will be no mystery as to the guilty party if someone sees you exit). In the absence of an

air-freshening spray, lighting a match afterward will usually get the job done.

(2) If forced to use a communal restroom, check other stalls to make sure you are alone. If possible, try to claim a handicapped stall (the Taj Ma-stall).

(3) If you are not alone and can no longer hold on, employ one of several techniques to mask the impending noise. The exaggerated cough/sneeze and continuous flush tactics are most effective, as is implementation of the Life Raft (see page 47). Also, be sure that your staff photo ID is not hanging off of your pants for the next-stall-neighbor to clearly identify who you are.

(4) *Always* employ a courtesy flush to minimize odor. A proper courtesy flush is executed immediately upon initiation of the bowel movement to minimize escape of noxious odors.

(5) Wash your hands thoroughly before returning to work. If you don't, the rumor mill will start turning and you will forever be "that guy" in the minds of your coworkers.

Poobiquitous

Synonyms: *Perpetual Poo, Poofinity, Stool Seepage*

A couple of loose, watery bowel movements after bad fast food is one thing; continuous seepage of stool from your rectal area is another. Despite moving their bowels several times a day, people suffering from Poobiquitous frequently discover their undergarments soiled with stool. The initial reaction upon finding yourself in this situation is to assume a hasty cleanup is to blame. When adoption of a more aggressive wiping protocol fails to stem the tide of liquid stool emerging from your rectum, you resort to placing wads of toilet paper in your underwear, hoping that this poo-in-perpetuity will soon cease. Ultimately, you question: Why the sudden, ceaseless seepage and how can it be stopped?

Dr. Stool says: Poobiquitous indicates the presence of a perianal fistula, an abnormal connection between the intestines and the skin surrounding the anus. In laymen's terms, this means that stool is coming out of your skin. Normally, stool is held in our rectum by contraction of the anal sphincter, a muscular valve that allows us to hold onto stool until a convenient time and place. Inflammation in the bowel, most commonly due to Crohn's disease, can cause the intestinal tract to erode into the perianal skin. This passageway allows stool to bypass the anal sphincter and results in continuous and untimely stool seepage. Historically, fistula treatment required surgery, but aggressive medical therapy with immunosuppressive drugs can now lead to healing in a majority of patients.

Nuggets

The consumption of yogurt can help with mild forms of diarrhea caused by antibiotics. Yogurt contains active bacterial cultures that help to "repopulate" the GI tract with colon-friendly organisms that may have been wiped out by our high-powered antibiotics.

THE OPPOSITE OF TALKING OUT OF YOUR BUTT

In rare cases of intestinal obstruction, it is possible to vomit poo. Most cases of bowel blockage occur in the small intestine (before poo is formed), but when the problem occurs in the large intestine and fecal matter cannot make its way out via the rectum, it travels in reverse into the upper GI tract and exits via the mouth. Treatment of this rare condition is almost always surgical in nature.

Doo You Know
The average individual can expect to see meal remnants in their stool thirty to forty hours after eating. Knowing your transit time may be useful if you are suffering from severe constipation or other gastrointestinal problems such as bloating. Perform a home transit test by simply downing a bowl of corn (or other colorful, insoluble fiber-rich food) and start your stopwatch!

Itchy Poo

Synonyms: *Scratch and (Don't) Sniff Stool, Prickly Poo*

Everyone, at some point, has had an uncontrollable, irrepressible urge to scratch the anal region after having a bowel movement. The urge to itch commonly comes as we lie in bed at night, sometimes during sleep itself. For most, this sensation will quickly pass within a day or two. For others, the desire to grab the nearest emery board and go at it persists for weeks and months. When occurring at night, this condition can interfere with restful sleep and leave nighttime scratchers tired and sluggish the next morning. When occurring during the day, the anal scratching will no doubt offend classmates, colleagues, and passersby. Public humiliation aside, anal itching can cause underwear to become stained and fingers to smell. If a quick change in your diet and laundry detergent doesn't offer relief, it's time to do yourself (and others) a favor and walk yourself, hands firmly in your front pockets, to the nearest doctor.

Dr. Stool says: The most common causes of perianal itching are medications (especially antibiotics), chemical irritants (laundry detergents, lotions), overly aggressive wiping, hemorrhoids, and a pinworm called *Enterobius vermicularis*. The itching associated with this pinworm infection is especially fierce at night when the female parasites emerge from the anal canal to lay ten thousand or so eggs on the perianal skin. These eggs cause severe irritation to the area, leaving the unsuspecting host no choice but to scratch away, thereby transferring eggs to the hands where they can be spread to others.

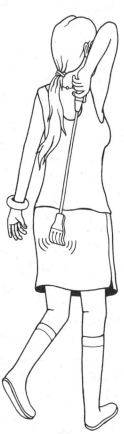

POO PURGE:
POO AS A WEAPON IN THE FIGHT AGAINST OBESITY

We live in a society where there is a lot of pressure to look thin. Magazines are filled with skinny models and there is no shortage of fad diets promising to help you lose weight fast. While some people maintain a disciplined workout regimen and commit to a healthy diet, others seek easier alternatives to lose weight. It should come as no surprise that many of these alternative weight-loss options involve the manipulation of one's GI system.

Poo Purge I: Cutting Weight

The practice of "cutting weight," which involves the use of laxative medicines to rapidly shed pounds, has long been employed in competitive sports such as wrestling. These medicines can cause the evacuation of large quantities of fecal material and water resulting in one to two pounds of rapid weight loss, an amount often sufficient to allow competition in a lower weight class. The main danger with this type of weight-loss method is the potential for dehydration and electrolyte abnormalities which, if severe, can lead to heart and kidney problems.

Poo Purge II: Orlistat

Interference with the body's ability to digest the foods we eat is a more aggressive strategy for weight loss employed by medications such as orlistat. Orlistat inhibits the activity of pancreatic lipase, an enzyme which digests the fat we consume in our diets. The end result of taking this medication is that the bucket of fried chicken never makes its way onto our hips. Sounds great, doesn't it? Ahh, but the grease must go somewhere. This is where poo comes in (or rather, goes out). The undigested fat remains in the intestinal tract and is eliminated in our feces, creating a yellow, glistening, foul-smelling stool that floats on the toilet surface (picture an oil spill in the ocean). In the case of orlistat, diarrhea is not a side effect—it is the *primary* effect. It's how the medicine works. For some, greasy, smelly poo is a small price to pay for the ability to have their cake (and lose it too).

Poo Purge III: Gastric Bypass

Stomach-stapling surgery, also known as gastric bypass, is the most extreme shortcut to achieving weight loss through something other than regular exercise and a healthy diet. The two basic objectives of this operation are to (1) make the stomach smaller and (2) rearrange the intestines so that a large portion of it never comes in contact with food (the "bypassed" segment). The end results are that (1) we eat less and (2) we absorb less of the food we eat. This surgery is remarkably effective, with most patients losing one to two hundred pounds in the first couple of years!

The effect on poo? Diarrhea used to be common following older procedures which bypassed larger portions of the small intestine (the small intestine is primarily responsible for absorbing nutrients) but is uncommon with today's procedures. In fact, due in part to the surgery's effects on the nerves that stimulate intestinal movement, constipation is more the norm in the postoperative period. Still, a particular complication with the very technical name "dumping syndrome" can occur in some patients. After surgery, the smaller stomach pouch empties its contents more quickly into the small intestine, which can cause bloating and watery diarrhea. Simple dietary modifications will usually relieve symptoms.

Doo You Know

Countless numbers of individuals with unexplained bloating, flatulence, and diarrhea need look no further than their daily choice of beverage to obtain relief from their symptoms. Sodas, with their sky-high levels of high-fructose corn syrup, are not so quietly causing an epidemic of irritable bowels in patients with undiagnosed fructose intolerance.

Gummy Poo

Synonyms: *Chewy Poo, Dubble Bubble Double, Duicy Fruit, Chewels Stools, Bubblicious Butt*

It turns out that one of life's simplest pleasures, chewing gum, can have unintended and untoward side effects on the GI tract. We have all been duly warned of the risks of swallowing gum (see Chapter Four's exposé on page 104), but it turns out that chewing a lot of gum (even if you spit it out) can cause abdominal distress. The culprit here is the artificial sweetener sorbitol, also known as glucitol, an ingredient commonly found in sugarless chewing gum. Sorbitol is poorly absorbed by the intestines and thus passes through to our colon where it has two main effects. First, it is fermented by bacteria to produce gas (thus causing bloating and cramping); and second, it actually works as a laxative by sucking water into the intestinal tract (hence, diarrhea). In fact, sorbitol is occasionally used as a laxative *treatment* for constipation.

Dr. Stool says: How much gum do you have to chew before things get bad? Usually a dose of more than ten grams of sorbitol per day is required to cause significant GI symptoms, and most people can tolerate up to fifteen grams per day. A typical stick of gum has 1.25 grams of sorbitol, so most people would have to chew a pack a day to get significant symptoms.

Nuggets

Postoperative ileus *is a common condition occurring after abdominal surgeries (appendectomies, C-sections, etc.) in which the bowel gets "stunned" into silence. A recent study showed that patients who chewed gum for fifteen minutes three times a day recovered bowel function faster and left the hospital sooner than patients who did not. Chewing gum apparently tricks the body into thinking that food is on its way, causing the brain to send signals which jump-start the intestines.*

THE HUE OF POO

• **Brown:** Stool's usual brown color is due to the presence of a compound called stercobilin, which is formed when the bacteria in our colon digest bile. Most daily variation in stool color is due to the dietary intake of various foods and medications. However, changes in stool color that persist for longer periods of time can be a sign of an underlying gastrointestinal disorder.

• **White:** Sometimes occurring after consumption of barium (the chalky stuff you drink before getting an X-ray or CT scan), white, or albino-looking, poo can also be caused by a blockage in the bile ducts or by various types of liver disease. This poo is rare and typically develops slowly over days to weeks (sometimes with a simultaneous darkening of the urine, see Gravy Train, p. 28). When it comes to poo, white is not right and a visit to your doctor is a must.

• **Black:** Stool sometimes diverges from its usual brown color and emerges as a dark black shade. This can be caused by foods that are high in iron (or iron pills), bismuth compounds (e.g., Pepto-Bismol), or blood (from higher up in the digestive tract).

• **Green:** When you expect to see a brown poo in the toilet, but instead are startled by a solid green log, there are two typical culprits: diet or infection. Green leafy vegetables such as spinach are the main dietary culprits of green poo. Green poo can also represent a gastrointestinal infection, especially with a bacterium called *Clostridium difficile*. Infection with this bug typically occurs after a course of antibiotics is taken for some other infection and can range in severity from mild to life-threatening. Treatment requires administration of a different type of antibiotic.

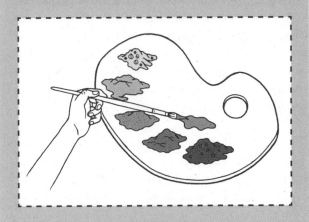

• **Red:** Red poo can be a sign of something as dangerous as blood in your lower digestive tract, or a result of something as innocuous as a heavy helping of beets. Any sighting of red poo (not preceded by eating beets) should be followed by a quick visit to the physician. Doctors may recommend a colonoscopy, a procedure which allows physicians to view the inside of the colon.

• **Yellow:** We all know that poo should be brown and pee should be yellow. Sometimes, however, the body produces a yellow-hued poo, leaving us to wonder why. Like most changes in the hue of poo, long-lasting perturbations are most worrisome. The main cause of yellow poo is the presence of fat in the stool, which occurs when dietary fats can't be digested by the body. This produces a yellow, glistening, floating stool indicating a problem with the small intestine, pancreas, or liver.

♨ Nuggets

The earliest documented use of enemas is found in the Egyptian Ebers Papyrus from 1500 B.C. Egyptians believed that all disease was caused by an excess of food and looked to enemas as a way to cleanse the system. In prerevolutionary France, enemas were used to cure a variety of ills and were even performed on a daily basis after dinner. Lore has it that Louis XIV was a fan of the practice, with some historians estimating that he received upward of two thousand enemas in his lifetime.

PREGNANT PAUSE

Irregularity is a regular phenomenon for pregnant women. GI discomfort in pregnancy can be attributed to two things. First, high levels of the hormone progesterone cause the muscles in the GI tract to relax and become sluggish. This slows intestinal movement and is the main reason why pregnant women suffer from constipation. Second, as pregnancy progresses, the growing uterus puts direct pressure on the bowels, thereby impeding their normal activity and further worsening constipation.

Increased dietary fiber and water, along with regular activity, is sufficient to ease constipation in most pregnant women. Stool softeners and gentle laxatives can also offer relief but should be taken only if symptoms persist. You can rest assured that the discomfort you are feeling, and the sounds and smells you are releasing, have no affect on your baby. While your spouse and coworkers may be suffering, your baby is impervious to your digestive distress.

Poo-nami

Synonym: *Baby Blowout*

Diaper technology has improved over the decades, but there has yet to come an innovation that can suppress the Poo-nami. While most baby poos can be contained by a diaper, there are instances when nothing can stop the poo from exploding beyond the confines of a diaper, up the baby's back, and down his or her legs. Dealing with Poo-namis is just one of the many challenges of parenthood.

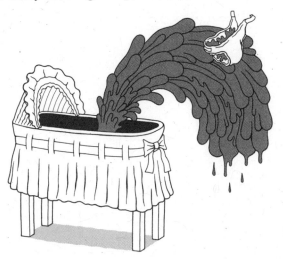

Dr. Stool says: Ill-fitting diapers are the most common cause of the dreaded Poo-nami. New parents who are inexperienced in proper diaper application techniques often suffer their share of Poo-namis during the first few months of parenthood. Poo-namis also tend to occur during bouts of diarrhea, most commonly due to rotavirus infection.

It is quite normal for infants to have explosive, liquid bowel movements in the first few months of life. This occurs because stool is frequently expelled simultaneously with gas. When stools become very frequent and voluminous, diarrheal illnesses such as rotavirus infection may be to blame.

LET'S GET READY TO RUMBLE!

Sometimes you can sense it coming. What starts out as an innocent murmur eventually builds into an all-out rumbling heard clear across the room. You knead at your stomach and attempt occasional throat-clearing or paper shuffling as a means to mask the sound, timing these actions to the predicted onset of the next wave, but, alas, you are helpless to stifle these gastric reverberations.

Borborygmi is the technical term given to this rumbling noise which emanates from the abdomen.

Its physiologic purpose is *not* to tell us when to eat but rather to sweep the intestines clear of debris left over from the prior meal. Called the "intestinal housekeeper," the MMC, or migrating motor complex, is a massive, wave-like intestinal contraction which begins in the stomach and ends in the large intestine. During periods of fasting, the MMC occurs every ninety minutes or so and rapidly transports gas, fluid, and solid debris down the GI tract (it is the gas movement which causes noise). Since the MMC only occurs in between meals, the rumbling it produces has come to signify hunger.

Borborygmi are a consequence of normal GI tract functioning and, thus, rarely signify disease. Certain medical conditions in which intestinal gas production may be increased, such as maldigestion (i.e., lactose intolerance) and bacterial overgrowth, have been associated with increased stomach rumbling.

Chapter Three:

The Gas We Pass

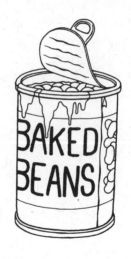

Just as everybody poops, everyone farts. In fact, while poo can come once or twice a day, flatulence can be an hourly event for some. Flatulence, like poo, has endured millennia in society's outhouse as another bodily process to be shunned and stifled, leaving us to wonder what could be so objectionable about the simple act of releasing air from the anus. Is it the obtrusive tooting sound generated during flatus's expulsion? Its repulsive rotten-egg aroma? Or were farts doomed from day one, done in by their relationship to poo, the bigger and bolder member of the excrement family?

Lighten up.

Smell the roses.

Let loose (just a little).

The time has come to give flatulence some long overdue airtime.

FLATOLOGY 101

Much of our flatal knowledge comes from the work of flatology pioneers, hardworking men and women who devoted their careers to the study of intestinal gas. These scientists determined the amount and composition of the gas we pass by analyzing flatulence collected in bags hooked up to volunteers' rectums. Talk about all guts and no glory . . .

This tireless and odoriferous work determined that farts are mostly nitrogen gas but also include a smattering of carbon dioxide, hydrogen, and, of course, glorious methane. The relative concentrations of these gases is determined simply by where the gas comes from. Swallowed air is high in nitrogen (nitrogen is the most abundant gas in the atmosphere), whereas intestinal gas produced, say, after consuming a bowl of black bean chili, will be high in carbon dioxide, hydrogen, and methane.

The average person expels between 400 and 2,400 cubic centimeters of flatus per day, divided into, on average, fourteen distinct emissions, or farts. Yes, that's right—quiet or loud, smelly or not, the average human farts more than a dozen times per day (and night). Flatus passage sometimes occurs inadvertently, say during a fit of coughing or sneezing, but on other occasions can be voluntarily produced by tensing the abdominal muscles and relaxing the anal sphincter. Unlike poo, flatus has no form so its derangements are broadly grouped into those of sound, smell, quantity, and circumstance.

Doo You Know

The Major Components of Human Farts Are:

- Nitrogen: 20 percent to 90 percent
- Carbon dioxide: 10 percent to 30 percent
- Hydrogen: 0 to 50 percent
- Oxygen: 0 to 10 percent
- Methane: 0 to 10 percent

The Explosion

Synonyms: *The Bullhorn, Air Show, Sonic Boom, Rolling Thunder*

Rarely heard in public due to societal constraints, the Explosion is characterized by its deafening sound, likened by some to the roar of a lion, by others to the revving of a jumbo jet engine. This deafening expulsion offers particular satisfaction as it usually indicates the release of highly pressurized gas. The decompression can leave you feeling light on your feet, while the raucous sound can bring about hearty congratulations (in the right company, of course).

A fart's loudness is determined by two main factors: the gas's volume and/or pressure, and the aperture through which it passes. Simply put, the greater the gas pressure and/or volume and the smaller the opening of the anal canal, the louder the fart. This association can be expressed mathematically through the following equation:

$$\text{FL (fart loudness)} \approx \frac{\text{Gas}_{\text{volume}} \text{ x Gas}_{\text{expulsion pressure}}}{\text{Anal canal diameter}}$$

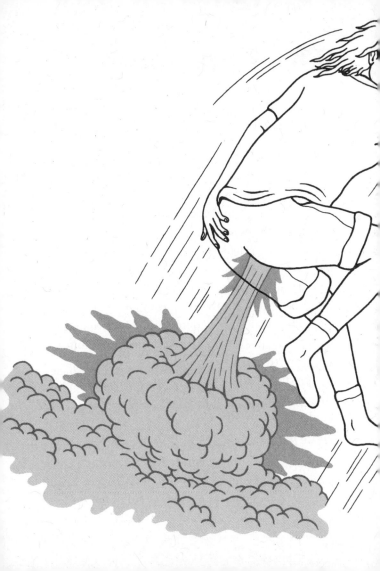

Gas volume is determined by two main factors: how much air we swallow and what we eat. All of us unconsciously swallow air as we go about our daily lives. Aerophagia, or excessive air swallowing, typically occurs in people who continuously chew gum or consume a large volume of carbonated beverages. The resultant intestinal buildup of nitrogen-rich gas is typically released by belching, but some of this gas finds its way down the GI tract for a backdoor exit.

A more likely cause of increased gas volumes is the consumption of indigestible carbohydrates found in foods such as chickpeas, cabbage, beans, brussels sprouts, broccoli, onions, and even red wine. These flatogenic foods evade digestion in the small intestine and thus make their way to the colon, where they undergo fermentation by intestinal bacteria. As part of the digestion process, these bacteria let off varying concentrations of carbon dioxide, hydrogen, and methane gas. The precise amount of each gas is dependent on the specific types of bacteria residing in the colon. Contrary to popular belief, only a third of us have the "right" bacteria to produce significant amounts of methane during this digestion process.

Gas expulsion pressure is dependent on the amount of gas to be expelled, but can also be affected by the strength of our abdominal muscle contractions. Abdominal muscle contraction (bearing down) forces stored gas out in a rapid, highly pressurized fashion.

Anal canal diameter: Think of the anal canal as Mother Nature's flute. The sound generated by a fart is dependent on the amount of reverberation it generates while passing through the anal corridor. The smaller the opening, the greater the reverberation and the louder the sound. Some gifted souls have an almost magical control over the size of their anal aperture and can willfully alter the intensity, duration, and pitch of their flatus. Structures like hemorrhoids, which protrude into the anal canal, dial up a fart's volume by rendering flow more turbulent.

Dr. Stool says: Most individuals with explosive flatus suffer from an increased amount of intestinal gas production. (We are assuming that most non-fraternity-dwelling people refrain from intentionally amplifying their flatulence by forcibly "expelling it." A careful dietary history will often reveal the responsible gas-producing food(s). Dairy products are a common culprit in those with lactose intolerance. If elimination of milk doesn't do the trick, try avoiding a few common accomplices (see "Flatogenic Foods" below). A quick glance will reveal that many gas-forming foods are plant-based; humans lack the ability to fully digest these foods, thereby leaving ample leftovers for the gas-producing bacteria in our large intestine.

FLATOGENIC FOODS

- Onions
- Lactose
- Beans
- Brussels sprouts
- Prunes
- Lentils
- Molasses
- Broccoli
- Coffee
- Apricots
- Wheat germ, oats, barley
- Chickpeas
- Cabbage
- Red wine
- Eggplant
- Dark beer

After eliminating all dairy and other flatogenic foods from your diet, if your body still produces Explosion farts, try stifling the sound by adopting techniques that will relax the abdomen (deep breathing is one such tactic). Experienced stiflers will actually suck in the abdominal wall in an attempt to decrease the force with which air is expelled. Whatever your tactics, avoid the urge to constrict your anal sphincter: remember, the smaller the opening, the louder the noise. Farting through a tight sphincter can make it seem as though you just tooted on a kazoo. Instead, try slowly releasing the air by gradually relaxing the anal sphincter over a few seconds.

Toots

The nineteenth-century French "fartiste," Joseph Pujol, better known by his stage name, "Le Pétomane," or "fart maniac," had the remarkable talent of being able to fart at will. His tricks included playing the flute with his anus and farting to blow out birthday candles stationed several yards away. He also had the ability to re-create animal sounds and typically opened acts with his own unique rendition of the French national anthem.

Morning Thunder

Synonyms: *Wake-up Call, Revelry, The Rooster*

This rumbling and resonant riptide of flatus heralds the beginning of a new day. Air passage typically occurs within thirty minutes of awakening, and if your partner or roommate happens to be asleep, the conch-like bellowing sound is sure to wake them. Admittedly not the most soothing way to be awakened, having a roommate with potent and predictable Morning Thunder does have the advantage of precluding the need for an alarm clock. In addition to its typical deep, reverberating sound, these early AM emissions are long in duration, easily lasting three to four seconds. Thankfully, this flatus is all bark and no bite; Morning Thunder's odor is classically benign.

Dr. Stool says: Morning Thunder is the result of an increase in the colon's muscular contractions which occur upon awakening. We all pass small amounts of gas while we sleep, but for most of the night, our colons are resting quietly. Upon awakening, our colonic activity

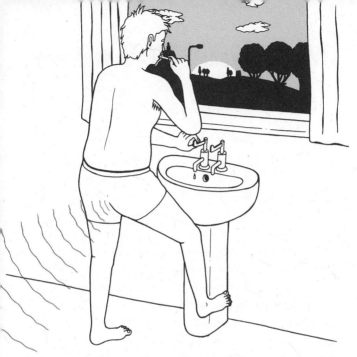

increases dramatically, causing rapid propulsion of fecal matter and gas along the length of the colon to the rectal area. These tidal wave–like movements called HAPCs, or high-amplitude propagating contractions, account for the need to break wind before we breakfast. Some individuals experience mild abdominal discomfort as gas is rapidly propelled down the colon, but quickly achieve relief with this early morning decompression.

DUTCH OVEN

When someone who is lying awake in bed farts under the sheets, then pulls the sheets over the head of their unsuspecting partner, it is called giving him or her a Dutch Oven. While a Dutch Oven is often seen as a cruel, juvenile act, openly farting in front of a partner signifies the development of an unwavering trust (or over-familiarity) in a relationship. The Dutch Oven is an extreme form of the Honeymoon's Over Fart, a close cousin of the Honeymoon's Over Poo. There is some debate as to whether the open pooing or farting milestone comes first in the natural progression of a relationship. One thing is certain, however: the honeymoon is most certainly over for couples that exchange Dutch Ovens.

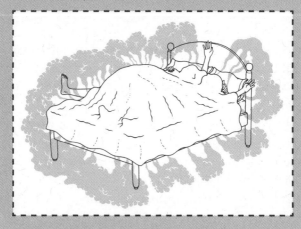

Doo You Know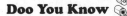

While we are peacefully sleeping, dreaming of vacations on the beach or strolls through the park, we are also farting. Turns out that while we are resting peacefully in bed, our anal sphincter muscles also relax, becoming weak and flaccid during sleep. The average number of nocturnal farts is unknown but estimates range between five and ten small, imperceptible releases.

Frequent Farter

Synonyms: *Status Flatus, Gas Leaker*

Fourteen episodes of flatulence a day may seem like a lot to the average person, but for Frequent Farters, fourteen farts would be a fortunate *hourly* total. As if every meal were laden with black beans and cabbage smothered in a cream sauce, these individuals cannot help but produce large amounts of foul-smelling flatus. Their rectums function much like a piston engine, with each rhythmic opening and closing of the anal sphincter being accompanied by the release of voluminous amounts of methane and hydrogen sulfide. As a means of survival, these individuals learn to modulate flatal volume and showcase a remarkable ability to stifle the sound of even the most pressurized emissions. Unfortunately, they lack the ability to regulate odor and thus become the most common perpetrators of the Silent But Deadly (see page 87). When spending time with a Frequent Farter, you don't need a rhyme to know who did the crime.

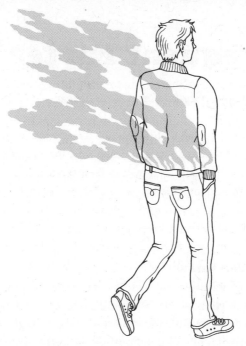

Dr. Stool says: The problem here is similar to what is seen with the Explosion (see page 74)—excessive production of intestinal gas—but in this case the situation is more chronic in nature, and dietary modification alone is often unsuccessful in correcting the problem. Intestinal bacteria produce virtually all the carbon dioxide, hydrogen, and methane found in farts. In some individuals, the number of gas-producing bacteria in the small intestine increases beyond healthy levels, resulting in abdominal bloating and increased flatulence. This condition, called bacterial overgrowth, can occur for a variety of reasons and is easily diagnosed by a simple breath test which measures levels of hydrogen and methane gas in expired air. Treatment of bacterial overgrowth is with antibiotics aimed at restoring bacteria to their normal levels.

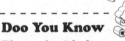

Doo You Know

Plagued with frequent flatus? Try simethicone, an over-the-counter medication used to treat increased levels of intestinal gas. It works by changing the surface tension of small air bubbles, allowing them to coalesce into large air bubbles, which are easier to pass. Farting frequency decreases as trapped air is more easily eliminated.

Silent But Deadly

Synonyms: *Stealth Bomber, Silent But Violent, Elephant in the Room*

We've all been there. Thirty minutes into the post-lunch staff meeting you begin to feel the rumblings of impending flatulence. Confident in your ability to release this air bolus in a covert fashion, you decide to liberate a small, seemingly harmless waft of air

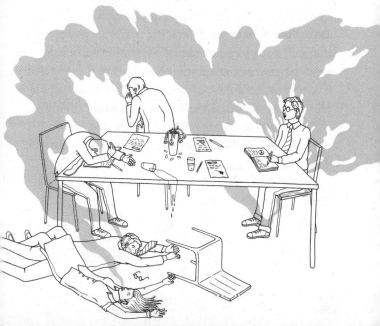

right there in the boardroom. You feel a sense of relief after the successful deployment and begin to grow proud of your accomplishment, marveling at your Zen-like ability to stealthily decompress your colon. Several seconds later, this braggadocio is replaced by sheer horror as you realize this ephemeral emission has taken on the aroma of a toxic waste dump. You may look around to see if there is a dog in the vicinity that you can blame. Ultimately, your fear is realized when colleagues begin shifting in their seats, lips firmly sealed, their faces scrunched in revulsion. You quickly feign the same sort of disgust, even mumbling to your neighbor, "Aw, man . . . who cut the cheese?" lest you be identified as the source of this most atrocious atmospheric contribution.

Dr. Stool says: The SBD is proof that while one can often estimate the volume of an impending fart, its odor can be infuriatingly unpredictable. In fact, a fart's toxicity has surprisingly little to do with its volume and everything to do with its concentration of hydrogen sulfide. Hydrogen sulfide, not the notorious methane, is the ingredient which lends flatus its distinctive eggy aroma. This gas is formed when bacteria ferment raffinose, a particularly potent carbohydrate found in brussels sprouts, cabbage, and other flatus-inducing plant-based products.

Toots

Some claim that standing on your head can help stifle flatus. This tactic presumably works by preventing gas from traveling through the intestinal tract to the rectum. Needless to say, the scientific community is skeptical of the headstand's efficacy.

The Victimless Crime

Synonyms: *Odorless Fart; No Harm, No Foul; Without a Trace*

The opposite of the SBD is the Victimless Crime. These odorless farts provide immediate physical relief from the gaseous pressure while the lack of aroma lends some equally important psychological relief. The Victimless Crime is like a delicious low-calorie dessert—all the pleasure with none of the guilt. Although highly desirable, especially for those working and living in close quarters, the odorless fart is also unpredictable. It should be noted that while claims of odorless flatus are plentiful, the truly odorless fart is indeed rare. Just as there are parents who believe their kid to be the most adorable on earth, there are equally delusional individuals who allege passage of unscented flatus as their norm.

 Dr. Stool says: Despite our efforts, newborn babies are the only humans who can truly perpetrate a victimless crime in the realm of flatulence. The newborn intestinal tract is devoid of bacteria (bacterial colonization begins immediately after birth) and therefore the majority of expelled air is composed of nitrogen and carbon dioxide, both odorless gases. Theoretically, aroma-free farts could be achieved by dietary elimination of all sulfide-producing foods and eradication of all intestinal bacteria through antibiotics or colonic "cleansing." As desirable as odorless flatulence may be, none of these strategies are advisable.

THE POST-MORTEM FARTS

Even after life ends, farting continues. Because gases build up in the body after death, corpses sometimes fart, startling morticians.

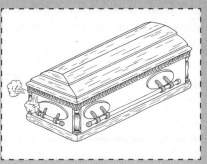

Smoke Signal

Synonyms: *The Sentinel, Opening Act, The Warning Shot, A-poo-tizer*

Seemingly just another fart upon deployment, the Smoke Signal is noteworthy because of what it portends. Its release typically occurs thirty minutes to one hour after a meal and can vary in intensity from a spurt to an eruption. Its aroma, however, is consistently abhorrent and can initially cause the responsible party to fear that he has expelled more than just gas. It may even prompt a quick pat to the backside to ensure that no solid matter has inadvertently escaped. A dash to the loo quickly follows the conclusion of the Smoke Signal, leaving little doubt in the minds of onlookers as to the perpetrator of this especially pungent "Opening Act."

Dr. Stool says: The Smoke Signal is best thought of as foreshadowing, an evolution-ary advance that alerts the owner (and, sometimes, others nearby) of the need to take care of more serious business. The release of a Smoke Signal broadcasts to those around you of your need to poo. The abhorrent aroma is the result of its prolonged cohabitation with fecal material. Rich in odoriferous sulfides, the Smoke Signal smells identical to a freshly laid log of good ol' number two. Its aroma is far from pleasant, and while denial is the usual reaction, ignoring its call for action can be even more catastrophic.

AIRTIGHT UNDERWEAR

Chester Weimer received a patent in 1998 for airtight underwear that is lined with a charcoal filter. This garment supposedly lets you fart with impunity by absorbing the emitted noxious odors. Lest you decide to don this diaper and let loose in company, bear in mind that the device may absorb odors but will do nothing to block out sounds.

CROP DUSTING

Crop Dusting is a surreptitious act that can be performed out of malice or as a means to avoid being identified as the source of a particularly vile-smelling emission.

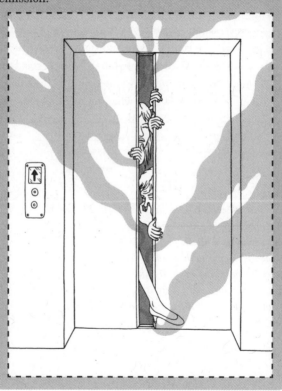

Crop Dusting is executed by precisely synchronizing flatal release with a brisk walk in the vicinity of a group of unsuspecting, distracted individuals, thereby leaving the abhorrent aroma in your wake. By the time the innocent bystanders catch wind of the stench, you are well on your way.

A much bolder variety of Crop Dusting is termed the Hot Box. The Hot Box, also known as an Air Raid or Elevator Expulsion, occurs when flatulence is released in a small, crowded, and contained space. There is no anonymity in a Hot Box, so when performing this devious act, be prepared to either apologize profusely or be mercilessly ridiculed and reviled.

Toots

While most cultures to this day shun those who pass flatus in public, it was the forward-thinking Roman emperor Claudius (10 B.C.–54 A.D.) who first legalized farting thousands of years ago over concern for people's health. By lifting the ban on farting at banquets, he was in line with the prevailing notion that retaining flatus could be harmful to one's health.

Veggie Fart

Synonyms: *Bean Bonanza, Going Green Gas, Tooting Tofu*

Vegetarians are known for tooting their own horns: they proclaim their compassion toward all living things and assert that their dietary practices are more environmentally friendly. Though annoying to some, this pride is justified when it comes to the function of the vegetarian gastrointestinal tract. Vegetarians have lower rates of constipation, hemorrhoids, diverticulosis, and colon cancer. But when it comes to flatulence, vegetarians are veritable gas-producing machines, blowing away their meat-eating compatriots with the frequency and volume of their expulsions.

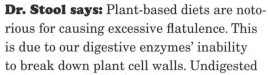

Dr. Stool says: Plant-based diets are notorious for causing excessive flatulence. This is due to our digestive enzymes' inability to break down plant cell walls. Undigested lettuce and broccoli make their way into the colon where bacteria devour them, liberating voluminous amounts of hydrogen and methane gas in the process.

But vegetarians may have the last laugh. True to their calm demeanor, it appears that they release flatulence in a more peaceful fashion. As we have discussed, the loudness of farts is inversely related to the size of the anal canal. The larger the opening, the softer the sound. Because vegetarians have larger, bulkier stools, they tend to have looser, more relaxed sphincters (though some would beg to differ), and hence, quieter flatulence. In addition, because meat protein is rich in sulfides, its consumption results in smellier flatus. So while vegetarians do fart more frequently, their flatus is quieter and less smelly.

Mile High Club

Synonyms: *High-Flying Farts, Airlift, Altitoots*

Sir Edmund Hillary and his Sherpa, Tenzing Norgay, are considered great men for their ability to overcome challenging conditions during their ascent to the top of the world's tallest mountain in 1953. The rugged terrain, ice storms, and bone-chilling temperatures must have paled in comparison to a lesser-known challenge of mountain climbing: flatulence. These heroic men almost surely suffered from excruciating abdominal pain resulting from the enormous quantity of gas which formed in their colons as they ascended Mount Everest. When it comes to flatulence, climbing to 29,000 feet is the equivalent of consuming bowl after bowl of black bean chili. A rarely discussed hazard of mountain climbing, the buildup (and release) of this expansive flatus can cripple even the most seasoned of climbers, making Hillary and Norgay's accomplishment even more remarkable.

Dr. Stool says: HAFE, or high-altitude flatus expulsion, is a gastrointestinal condition of increased flatus passage that occurs in people climbing to high altitudes. Higher altitudes mean lower atmospheric pressures, thereby causing intestinal gas to expand (physics reference: Boyle's Law), which results in intestinal distention and the need to pass flatus more frequently. HAFE becomes problematic when climbers ascend to altitudes above 11,000 feet. In a study of military recruits who were instructed

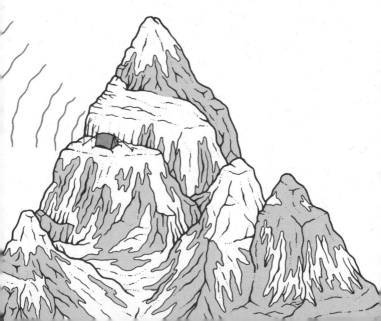

not to pass gas, scientists found that 110 milliliters of intestinal gas at sea level expanded to 500 milliliters at an altitude of 29,300 feet (about the height of Mount Everest). There is good news, however, among all this excess flatulence—most of the expelled air consists of carbon dioxide and is therefore relatively odorless. The physicians who first described this condition in 1981 characterized HAFE as a "significant inconvenience to those who prefer to hike in company."

Doo You Know

An Australian study found that men fart an average of fifteen times a day while women let loose a mere eight times a day. The study also concluded, however, that women's farts had higher sulfide content and smelled worse. Their scientific method? Subjects farted into an aluminum bag. The gas was then removed with a syringe and expelled into the nostrils of the eagerly awaiting judges.

FART PROUDLY

"Fart Proudly" is the title of a 1781 essay on flatulence written by Benjamin Franklin. In the text, Benjamin Franklin proposes, tongue in cheek, that the Royal Academy should use science to convert farts into something more agreeable to society.

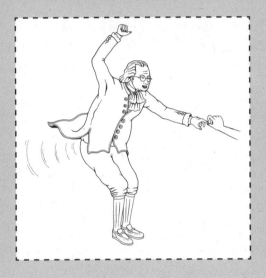

Chapter Four:

Bodily Myths Exploded

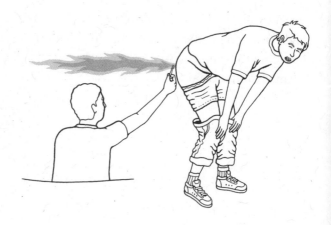

In the preceding pages, we have attempted to clarify many of the body's excremental dilemmas. This section will take stock of the most well-entrenched theories regarding our digestive and urinary systems to see if they hold water.

Many of us first encounter these anecdotes as young children. We wonder, from then on, whether these old wives' tales regarding the human body are based on sound medical knowledge or should be flushed down the toilet with the next bowel movement. Until now, these legends have escaped scrutiny while being indiscriminately passed down from one generation to the next. The time has come to bring clarity to the murky myths of the gastrointestinal tract.

Myth or Truth?

It takes seven years to digest chewing gum

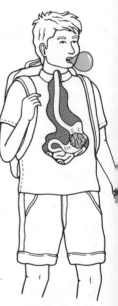

Dr. Stool says: While it is true that very few people are walking around with softball-sized, multicolored gumballs rolling around in their stomachs, the admonition against ingesting gum comes from the sound knowledge that the body lacks the ability to digest the rubbery base in chewing gum. Furthermore, this concept of a ball of undigested material in the stomach is called a bezoar and is a real medical entity first described thousands of years ago. A bezoar is simply a collection of undigested material that accumulates in the stomach. Usually seen in patients with a condition called gastroparesis in which the stomach's ability to empty food is severely impaired, a bezoar can also occur in healthy individuals due to consumption of indigestible substances. The most bezoar-genic food? Persimmons.

A particular bezoar known as trichobezoar is formed when individuals consume large quantities of their own hair. This can result in the formation of a hair ball and an honest-to-goodness medical condition called Rapunzel syndrome in which the hair ball causes stomach blockage. As our bodies lack the ability to digest hair, successful removal of this obstructing hair ball is achieved via endoscopic surgery.

Other substances that can form bezoars:

- Apples
- Celery
- Figs
- Sauerkraut
- Green beans
- Antacid medications
- And, yes, bubble gum

Don't fret, there is no need to throw away the rest of the celery and fig salad you were savoring. Consumption of these items (including bubble gum) rarely results in bezoar formation in people whose stomachs are functioning normally. So, unless you have had stomach surgery in the past or have been diagnosed with stomach-emptying problems, don't worry too much about bezoars. But just to play it safe, let's go ahead and hold the persimmons.

Myth!

Drinking urine is good for your health

Dr. Stool says: The thought of using a bodily waste product as a means to promote health may initially seem ridiculous. But there is a burgeoning movement in the West to harness the power of urine therapy, known as shivambu in the Indian ayurvedic tradition, to enhance the immune system and prevent disease. Former Indian Prime Minister Morarji Desai was one of the most famous proponents of urine therapy. He attributed his longevity (he lived to the ripe age of ninety-nine) to his daily intake of urine.

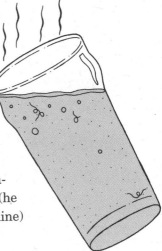

Urine consists of 95 percent water and 2.5 percent urea, with the remaining 2.5 percent a mixture of minerals, salts, hormones, and enzymes. It is also sterile. While there is no conclusive medical evidence of health benefits from drinking urine, the consumption of small amounts of one's own urine is unlikely to have serious adverse effects. Those taking medications, however, should resist the urge to pour themselves a tall frosty one, as their urine may contain harmful chemicals.

Eager to see if your golden stream can become your fountain of youth? Urine therapy proponents advise collecting midstream urine from the morning's first void.

Truth! *

*According to some.

Myth or Truth?

It is possible to light farts on fire

Dr. Stool says: Childhood stories about lighting farts are ubiquitous. Lore has it that iridescent blue and orange rays of light can be created by holding a lighter up to the rectum while flatus is released. Flatus is composed of varying concentrations of five major gases, two of which—hydrogen and methane—are flammable. When present in sufficient quantities and exposed to an open flame, flatus undergoes combustion and can indeed produce a colorful display. The chemical reactions are listed below:

Hydrogen: $2H_2S + 3O_2 \rightarrow 2SO_2 + 2H_2O$
Methane: $CH_4 + 2O_2 \rightarrow CO_2 + 2H_2O$

The most common color resulting from fart ignition is orange (although virtually all colors have been reported) created during combustion of hydrogen sulfide gas. A fart's color is determined by the specific types of bacteria and their relative

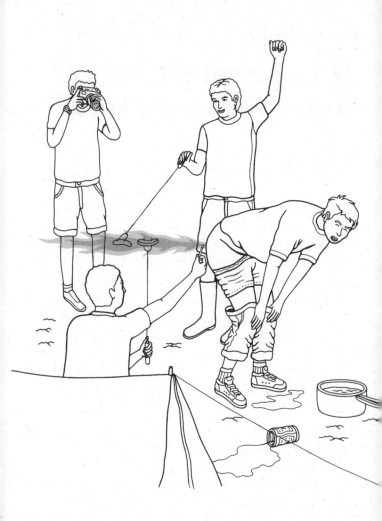

concentrations in the colon. Before you rush out to buy a bushel of baked beans and a lighter to create your own flatal fireworks, remember that serious bodily injury can occur. Although soundly rooted in science, this is one experiment not to be taken lightly.

Truth!

BLUE FART

Like the pink diamond, blue farts are rare (and highly coveted). The blue hue is created by the expulsion of methane gas, produced by only one-third of human beings. Surprisingly, the rest of us lack the necessary genetics and bacterial composition to produce methane gas, thereby limiting our flatal color spectrum to orange and yellow.

The menstool cycle: Men who live together poo on the same cycle

Dr. Stool says: After a few months of living together, women will begin synchronizing their menstrual periods. A similar phenomenon, which the *Urban Dictionary* has termed the "menstool cycle," has been observed in groups of men with regard to their stooling practices. Presumably, the once-a-weekers and three-times-a-dayers meet somewhere in between and begin to poo in unison. This can pose logistical problems in college frat houses where a single bathroom may be shared by a dozen guys. On a positive note, stooling synchrony can also lead to a greater sense of camaraderie.

Menstrual synchronization amongst women has been explained by the release of chemical messengers called pheromones. These scent molecules are detected by cohabitating women and somehow cause ovulation to occur at the same time of the month. Poo, too, emits its own unique blend of aromas, but they are admittedly universally unpleasant and unlikely to lure others into the bathroom (if anything, they are more likely to have the opposite effect). The more likely explanation for the menstool cycle is the shared pattern of eating and sleeping among housemates.

Simply put, we poo after we eat and we poo after we wake up. Movement of stool through the colon speeds up approximately thirty minutes after eating and almost immediately upon awakening in the morning. These physiologic principles of poo should apply equally to women, leaving us to wonder why this same poo synchrony is not seen in cohabitating females (or whether they just don't talk about it).

Truth!

Myth or Truth?

Sitting on the toilet for too long causes hemorrhoids

 Dr. Stool says: Hemorrhoids are enlarged veins in the anal canal that have a tendency to become irritated and bleed. They are formed from years of increased pressure, most commonly in constipated individuals who forcefully bear down in order to have a bowel movement.

Medical studies have found that if you spend an excessive amount of time on the toilet, you may be at risk for developing hemorrhoids (regardless of how smoothly you complete the deed). In fact, one study even found that hemorrhoids became smaller after patients stopped reading on the toilet! It seems that spending too much time on the toilet can be bad for your health.

Truth!

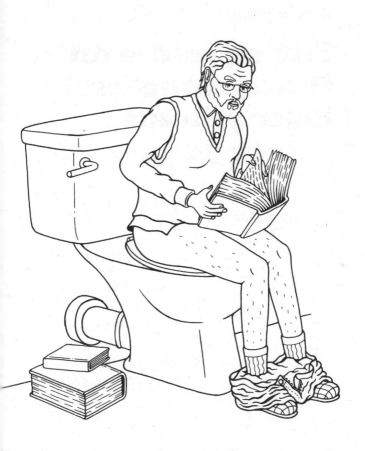

You should wait thirty minutes after you eat before swimming

Dr. Stool says: As kids, we counted the minutes after lunch until we could jump into the pool. On those hot summer days, thirty minutes could seem more like three hundred. Presumably, waiting thirty minutes would allow for adequate digestion of food and prevent vomiting once swimming commenced. Well, it turns out this half-hour respite between eating and swimming has no scientific basis whatsoever.

Studies show that it takes, on average, four hours to completely empty our stomachs. Food needs to be mixed with gastric juices and broken down into smaller particles prior to entering the small intestine (when the risk of vomiting with exertion is thought to be less). The thirty-minute moratorium on swimming makes little sense considering that over 90 percent of our hamburger and French fries would still be in the stomach at that point!

Some have argued that waiting 30 minutes after a meal to exercise will help prevent abdominal cramping. Blood diverted to our exercising muscles can theoretically decrease the amount of blood available to our intestinal tract and, thus, cause cramping. There is nothing to support, however, the firm 30-minute moratorium placed on exercise after eating. In fact, there is substantial evidence that light exercise after meals can help with the digestive process.

Myth!

Myth or Truth?

Peeing on your feet will get rid of athlete's foot

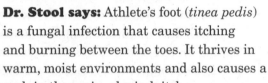 **Dr. Stool says:** Athlete's foot (*tinea pedis*) is a fungal infection that causes itching and burning between the toes. It thrives in warm, moist environments and also causes a similar rash in the groin, aka jock itch.

Peeing on your feet is a surprisingly effective way of treating mild cases of athlete's foot. Urine contains urea, a substance found in many over-the-counter athlete's foot treatments. The urea seems to work by making antifungal medications more effective (it somehow breaks up the dead skin and allows the drug to penetrate to where the fungi are hiding). The urea content in urine is low (2.5 percent) so you would have to soak your feet in urine to have a real impact, but, hey, at least it gives you an excuse to pee in the shower.

Truth!*

*Kind of.

Myth or Truth?

To survive extreme dehydration, drink your own urine

Dr. Stool says: Some people recommend drinking your own urine when stranded in the desert or on a life raft surrounded by salt water. In fact, there is anecdotal evidence of people surviving earthquakes trapped in rubble by drinking their own urine.

To determine the safety of drinking urine, remember two things: urine is 95 percent water (at least for the first few days of dehydration) and it is sterile. Our bodies need water to survive (we can go weeks without food), so urine is a surprisingly logical choice when no other hydration options are available. The jury is out on whether this practice is safe for more than a few days, as urinary concentration of harmful substances (e.g., urea) increases over time.

Truth!*

*At least for a few days.

Myth or Truth?

Your own poo doesn't stink

Dr. Stool says: We all know someone, maybe a significant other or a roommate, who exits the bathroom after dropping a deuce with his or her nose to the sky as if to say, "I've got nothing to hide." These individuals see no need for a courtesy flush and leave no lag time between poo deployment and flinging open the bathroom door. Some may even liken their excrement to various air freshener scents. Poo-pourri, anyone?

How rational people can fail to recognize that, *Yes, your dookie does stink,* is truly one of the great mysteries of poo. In fact, while most people don't emerge from the bathroom with reckless post-BM bravado, it is fair to say our poo smells worse to others than it does to us. How many times has your partner recoiled after walking into the stink chamber you unknowingly created?

Being able to detect poo's aroma would seem to be important from an evolutionary standpoint.

Serious ailments such as gastrointestinal bleeding and infections can often be sniffed out by changes in poo's smell. Why, then, has our sense of smell evolved in such a way as to sometimes render our own poo essentially odorless? This is one myth that will remain a mystery. Regardless, it is best to acknowledge the universal smelly nature of poo (yes, even your own) and do all that you can to protect your loved ones after the deed is done.

Myth!

Myth or Truth?

Holding in a fart is bad for you

Dr. Stool says: Ever since humans began living and working indoors, our ability to fart with impunity has been compromised. No longer can we let 'er rip without first ensuring our isolation. As a result, despite the discomfort, we sometimes elect to hold it in. Flatus retention is frequently associated with some transient abdominal distress, but it is only natural to wonder whether there is any serious downside to ignoring the body's urge to vent.

Some flatus experts have linked increasing rates of diverticulosis (outpouchings in the colon wall) to flatal retention. Holding air in the colon, they reason, increases intracolonic pressure, causing herniation and the formation of diverticula over time (like overinflating an old tire). No studies have proven this association but the rates of diverticulosis have been shown to be higher in industrialized countries where, presumably, office workers have greater pressure to suppress gaseous emissions.

Truth!*

*Possibly.

GLOBAL WARMING

While the effects of flatal retention on the human body remain unclear, there may be one good thing to come from a society of fart suppressors: less global warming! Methane gas makes up a small, but sizeable, proportion of gases emitted with each fart. Its ability to trap heat in the atmosphere makes it an important contributor to global warming. The importance of methane destruction in the fight against global warming is best demonstrated by the ongoing research dedicated to reducing the amount of methane found in cow flatulence by modifying their diets.

Peeing on a jellyfish sting will relieve the pain

Dr. Stool says: Jellyfish cause stinging by injecting an alkali-based fluid through little stingers called nematocysts. Some have claimed that urine's acidity can help neutralize the venom and relieve pain. In fact, normal urine is usually neutral (pH 7) or only slightly acidic and is probably only marginally effective for jellyfish stings. Dr. Stool recommends using a more acidic substance like vinegar (pH 2.5 or so) instead. While it may be inconvenient to carry a bottle of vinegar to the beach, pouring vinegar on your arm is a bit more socially acceptable than peeing on it.

Myth!

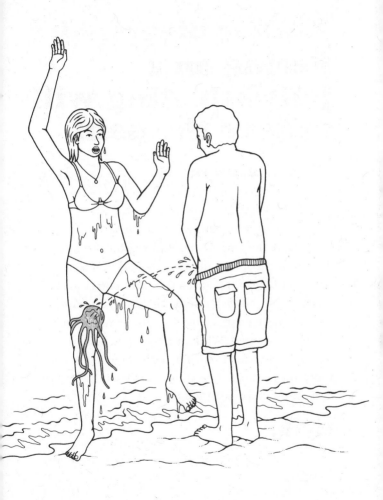

Author Biographies

Josh Richman met his coauthor while they were undergraduates at Brown University. Their shared fascination with the inner workings of the human body, along with their mutual appreciation of good fart jokes, brought them together to write this book. Josh holds an MBA from Stanford University and lives in the San Francisco Bay Area.

Anish Sheth, M.D., holds a medical degree from Brown University and is a gastroenterologist and Assistant Professor of Medicine at Yale University School of Medicine. After an eight-month hiatus from daily diaper changes, Anish is once again dealing with the all-too-frequent Poo-nami.

It's now safe to flush.